The doctor treats, the nature heals

How to treat hypertrophy of prostate by plants

Dr. Roger Billard

Edition Health by Plants

Table of Contents

INTRODUCTION

It's a Saturday. The weather is nice. We are in the village hall of a town hall of France. Mayor, in his ceremonial clothes of the big days, is celebrating a marriage. The happy couple is here, as well as a crowd of friends. But now our Mayor, while officiating in full solemnity, dignified and respectable before God and men, was suddenly seized by a down-to-earth concern: he suddenly had a pressing and irresistible desire to relieve himself. He tried to restrain himself, but nothing helped, he could not resist. If he did not find a solution, quickly, something was going to dribble from his pants, in full view of all the audience, and in front of the future newlyweds. Then, constrained, very contrite and sheepish, the Mayor mumbled a few words of excuse, interrupted the ceremony, and disappeared for five minutes, to go to the toilet.

What is the big problem of the Mayor?

Hey! Well, the Mayor was suffering from benign prostatic hypertrophy.

If you are between 40 and 90 years old, or more, or even less, you may also be concerned with the problem of benign prostatic hypertrophy (BPH). Around the world, about two out of every three men over the age of 50 are affected by BPH, and nearly one million people in France, of the same age group, are in this situation.

Specifically, all these people are faced with urges to urinate every hour, or even every half hour, with, in addition, a painful or uncomfortable urination. In penalty, these people, because of the BPH, can suffer serious problems of erection and thus of disturbed sexual life.

How to solve this problem?

Classical medicine offers treatments based on pharmacy and surgery that are expensive, sometimes leaving a legacy. In all cases, these treatments are not always effective.

Natural and alternative medicine, through plants, offers alternative treatments, the results of which are more and more convincing, and more and more used all over the world. It resorts to remote experiences in different parts of the world where plants, through their leaves, bark, flowers or roots, have been used with great success.

This book, after an overview of the organ of the prostate, the symptoms of benign prostatic hypertrophy and the standard treatments offered in health facilities, gives a detailed presentation of alternative treatments for the disease by plants and gentle methods.

1 - What is the prostate?

The prostate is an odd gland, a male genital organ, therefore present only in humans. Its function is to produce the prostatic fluid which represents about 30% of the sperm. The prostatic fluid fluidizes the sperm and serves as nutrients for the spermatozoa it protects, moreover It GIVES the sperm alkaline, which allows the spermatozoa to survive in the acidic environment of the woman's vagina.

The prostate is located below the bladder, behind the pubis, in front of the rectum. It surrounds, in its initial part, the urethra IS the canal by which the urine and the sperm are expelled. It is thus at the confluence formed by the urethra and spermatic ways. It is self wrapped in a connective tissue. Its volume increases from birth to puberty to be, for a healthy adult, the weight is between 20 to 25 g compare to the size of a ping-pong ball.

Figure N ° 1: Localization of the prostate in the human body

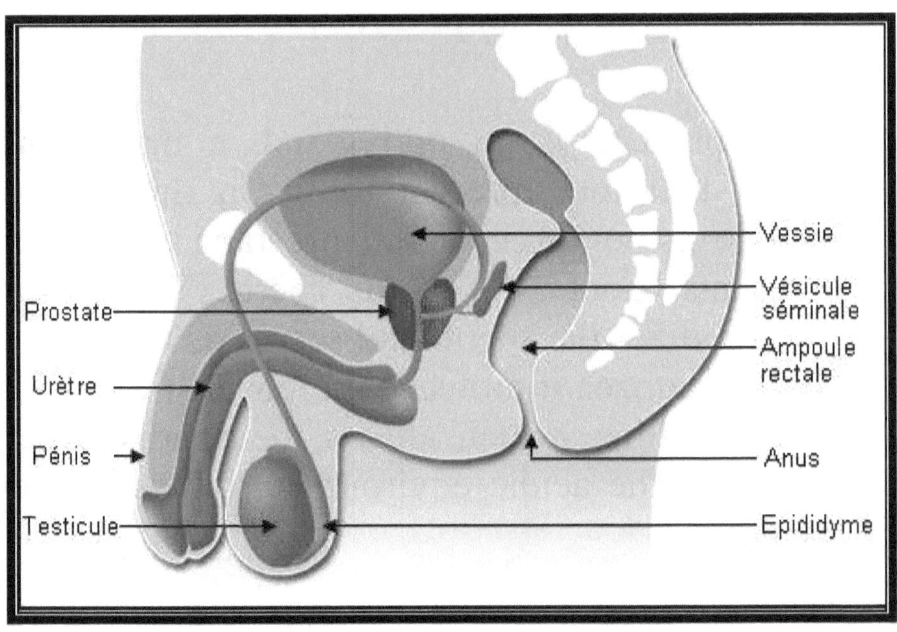

2 - What is Benign Prostatic Hypertrophy (BPH)

The prostate, from 40 years, begins to grow in humans. When its volume becomes important, it compresses the urethra and trouble the evacuation of the urine by this channel. This is called prostate adenoma, or hyperplasia, or hypertrophy of the prostate. This hypertrophy of the prostate is, in most cases, benign, it is called in this case "benign prostatic hypertrophy" (BPH). Benign because of the hypertrophied tissues that are not of cancerous nature, otherwise, it would be then question of malignant hypertrophy or cancer of the prostate. This hypertrophy is the result of proliferation of epithelial and stromal cells of prostatic tissue which is a part of the prostate called "transition zone" which is the seat of this anarchic multiplication of cells.

The three diagrams below show, successively:

- A bladder and a normal prostate;
- Asymptomatic microscopic lesions of the prostate;
-An urethra compressed by a hypertrophied prostate.

The risks of BPH are approximately 10% at age 30, 50% at age 60, and 90% at age 85 and older.

Figure N ° 2: Evolution of the volume of the prostate

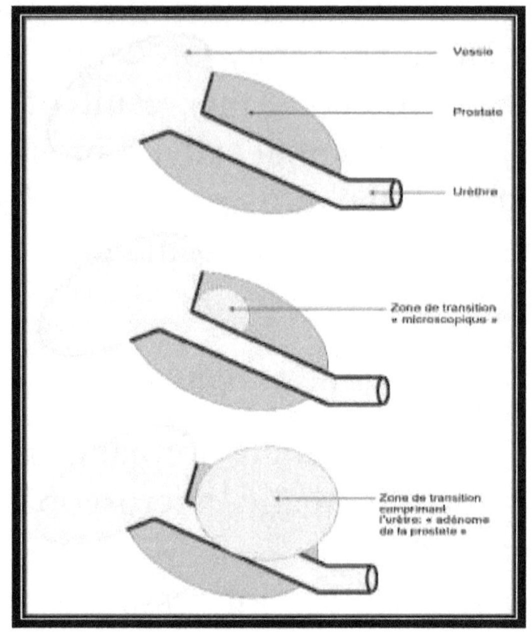

Source: P.-E. Briant, A. Ruffion; Reference: Prog Urol, 2009, 19, 4, 274-27

Figure N ° 3: Diagram of a normal prostate and a hypertrophied prostate

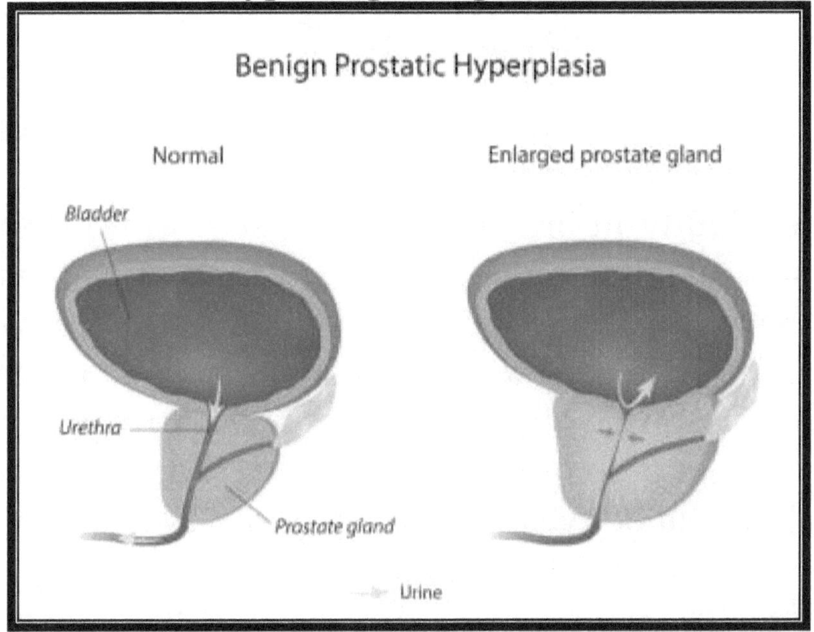

Source: Health, Nature, Innovation - In "Prostate, Natural Protocol"

3 - Life problems posed by benign prostatic hypertrophy

BPH causes different genes, or even several major problems in the daily life of man. The main ones are as follows.

- Problems related to urination: men, suffering from this evil, must frequently go to the toilet to relieve themselves, up to six or seven times a night, and even more during the day. This is very troublesome for sleep, for activities and for life in society. You are in the middle of a meeting, and you have to be away every hour to relieve yourself, which is not at all convenient. This discomfort is even accompanied by a difficulty in urinating, a slow start to urination, a weakness of the urinary stream that can even be jerky. The sick man is sometimes seized with an urge to urinate, while maybe, he is in his car, or in full working session with partners, and failing to go quickly to the toilet, he can urinate in his underwear. In addition, the evacuation of urine from the bladder is incomplete. This results a residue of urine that remains permanently in the bladder, which promotes the development of various bacteria that can cause inflammation and other diseases of the prostate. The problem can even go as far as the impossibility of urinating (urinary retention).

- Erection problems: The swelling of the prostate compresses the blood vessels that irrigate the penis and the sexual region. This causes difficulty in having a strong and persistent erection to allow vaginal penetration. To this can be added the difficulty of ejaculating. The sexual life of the couple is thus greatly disrupted and the harmony of the partners undermines.

- Complications: BPH can lead to serious complications such as:

- Impossibility to urinate: This happens when the pressure of the prostate is too strong to completely close the urethra, preventing the bladder from emptying its contents. The patient then feels severe pain. An urgent intervention is required in this case, with the need to place a probe to evacuate urine from the bladder. It should be noted, however, that these extreme cases are quite rare.

- Urinary stones: there may be mineral deposits in the bladder causing urinary stones, resulting in infections, as well as inflammation of the bladder wall, with impediment to urine evacuation.

- Distention of the bladder walls: The increased volume of the prostate can stretch the walls of the bladder and promote its early aging. It loses its strength and flexibility.

- Impairment of the kidneys: The kidneys may lose, over time, their ability to filter blood, because of the infections they are subject to caused by the permanent retention of urine in the bladder. This can lead to long-term renal failure.

CHAPTER 2:

THE TREATMENT OF BENIGN PROSTATIC HYPERTROPHY BY CLASSIC MEDICINE

The treatment of BPH by conventional medicine has many limitations and many adverse effects more or less troublesome.

We will review them, specifying the advantages and disadvantages of each.

1 - Treatment with synthetic drugs

Beta-sitosterol: Clinical trials conducted in 1999 showed that beta-sitosterol has positive results on the facilitation of urination (the ease of urination) but does not affect the reduction of the volume of the prostate. This product is available in pharmacy.

Alpha-blockers: The alpha-blockers used to treat BPH are doxazosin, terazosin, alfuzosin, tamsulosin and silodosin. These medications promote the flow of urine by relaxing the smooth muscles of the prostate and bladder neck. However, they have side effects including hypotension, fatigue, nasal congestion and ejaculation disorder.

Inhibitors of 5-α reductase: These drugs affect the volume of the prostate by inhibiting the production of the hormone responsible for the growth of the prostate. The results can last several years, but they have side effects: At the end of treatment, the symptoms of low libido and erectile dysfunction reappear. Depression has also been reported.

Anticholinergics: The anticholinergics used against BPH are oxybutynin, tolterodine and trospium chloride. They fight urinary incontinence. The effects are all very modest.

Inhibitors of Phosphodiesterase: Inhibitors of phosphodiesterase are mainly sildenafil, tadalafil and vardenafil. They would cure the symptoms of BPH, but in January 2013 in the UK, the National Institute for Health and Clinical Excellence did not recommend the use of these products for BPH due to lack of evidence provided by the manufacturer .

Surgery open or high: It is practiced for prostate volumes greater than 50 cm3. The surgical treatment consists of either a prostatectomy, that is the TOTAL removal of the prostate, or an adenectomy, that is a suppression of the only adenoma. This is done by the high route and is only considered in case of failure of the medical treatment and the radiological treatment. The surgical procedure can present many complications, namely:

- Urinary retention;
- The formation of blood clots in the bladder;
- Hemorrhages;
- Infection with microbial or bacterial agents;
- Retrograde ejaculation;
- Incontinence, most often transient;
- Narrowing of the diameter of the urethra.

Tran's rectal endoscopic resection or endo-urethral resection of the prostate (REUP): It is generally performed when the volume of the prostate is less than 50 mL (CM3). This involves removing the hypertrophied portion of the prostate by vaginally or naturally, maintaining the prostate envelope. To do this, we introduce a special endoscope called resistor in the urethra to remove small pieces of the prostate, until removing all the hypertrophied part of the organ. This intervention leads to a normalization of the urinary flow in 80% of the cases and to improve the symptoms in 90% of the cases.

The major disadvantage of this technique is retrograde ejaculation. That is, during orgasm, the sperm, instead of accumulating in the prostate and flowing through the urethra, accumulates in the bladder. This can cause infertility.

The complications that may occur during the operation are as follows:

- hemorrhages;
- The constitution of blood clot in the bladder;
- Incontinence.

The prostatic crevice incision: This involves making a Trans rectal incision of the bladder neck and the prostate. The goal is not to reduce hyperplasia but to reduce the existing resistance of the bladder. To do this, we use a resistor, not to resect the prostate, but to achieve one to two incisions on the prostatic urethra and on the bladder neck. This technique is used for prostate volumes not exceeding 30g. The major disadvantage is the retrograded ejaculation.

3 - Radiological treatment

These include interstitial radio frequency. It consists of introducing, under anesthesia, an endoscope comprising two antennas which is inserted into the prostatic tissue. The device then delivers a radiofrequency energy that causes necrosis lesions in the prostate. The major disadvantage of this technique is the irritation syndrome which can persist for several weeks. This technique is however less effective than surgical treatments.

4 - Laser Endoscopic Treatments

Those treatments consist of using an endoscope to introduce laser fibers into the prostate and then allow operating according to two techniques:
- Laser vaporization: High energy lasers are used to vaporize tissues. This technique is simple to control and is less hemorrhagic.
- Laser resection: This involves cutting the prostate endoscopic ally and sending the pieces into the bladder. A grinder is then introduced to grind the prostate pieces into

small fragments that can be removed by the urinary tract.

5 – Thermotherapy

Probes are placed in the urethra and in the rectum, and by means of a machine, microwaves producing heat are delivered. The effectiveness of this technique proved weak, which led to its abandonment.

6 – Intra-prostatic prostheses

It is a question of putting prostheses, temporary or definitively, in the urethra, to allow the flow of the urine.

CHAPTER 3:
TREATMENT OF BENIGN PROSTATIC HYPERTROPHY BY PLANTS AND NATURAL METHODS

1 - Ezee Flow Herbal Tea for Prostate

The Ezee Flow herbal tea for the prostate was developed by Nick Jerch, the founder of Bell Lifestyle.

This natural herb, consumed in the form of tea, is recommended for the natural treatment of benign prostatic hypertrophy.

Its healing properties are as follows:

- A significant reduction in the volume of the prostate;
- Resolving erection problems with a return to a fulfilling sex life by allowing normal and satisfying sex for both partners;
- Facilitation of urination by avoiding drip of urine and frequent and painful urination;
- A reduction in the frequency of urination by allowing restful nights;
- Restoration of urinary jet strength, increased urinary flow and complete urination.

Ezee Flow Herbal Tea was developed from twelve plants, including cranberry and chamomile.

Nick Jerch explains how he developed the product: "After a few experiments, I put together a mix of 14 different kinds of tea. After 3 days, each of the ingredients, mixed in different amounts, brought me the much desired relief. Friends who had to get up several times each night to go to the bathroom also tried it and were relieved just as quickly (one of them after 4 days, another after 5 days, and another could sleep all night without getting up after only 9 days). They were all delighted. Sleep interruptions can become a serious problem because you may not be able to go back to sleep. You are tired the next day and can hardly be productive for the entire duration of your work. As a bonus, everyone loves the aroma and taste of tea.

The instructions for use are as follows:

Take herbal tea on an empty stomach, that is, 30 minutes before meals, or two hours after meals. The herbal tea is packaged in sachets of a few grams that must be prepared as follows: Take a container and put a bag of Ezee Flow. Add five glasses of water, 25 cl glasses, or a total volume of 100 cl. Boil for ten minutes, then continue cooking over low heat for twenty minutes, then let cool and store in a thermos. The dosage of the intake is a glass of 25 cl of herbal tea prepared, twice a day, morning and evening, fasting, that is to say, 30 minutes before breakfast or 2 hours after, for the case of a catch in the morning, and 30 mn before the dinner or 2 hours after, for catch in the evening.

Depending on the size of the prostate, it may be necessary to follow the treatment for 2 to 3 months to have significant results.

This is for a cure. For maintenance treatment, after the expected results have been obtained, is a daily intake of one drink, always on an empty stomach.

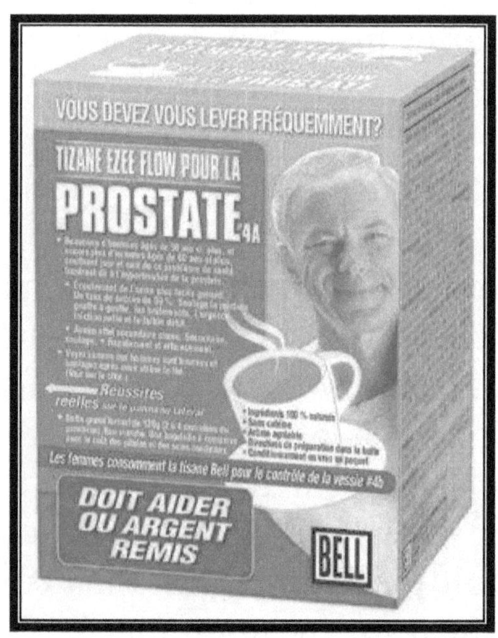

Figure N ° 4: A packaged box of Ezee Flow
herbal tea

The initiator of the product reports the following testimonials, from people who made use of the product:

Ronald St-Martin, St-Robert, QC: I found my happiness again. I started drinking your herbal tea, and in the days that followed, a slight improvement was noticed. After 4 weeks a relief of 90%. I am a happy man NOW. I got up 5 to 7 times a night in addition to regularly changing underwear. Now I get up 1 to 2 times a night and I do not have any problems with the flow. I wanted to write to you just to tell you that I am very satisfied because I refund my joy of living.

J. Marc Larrivé, Matane, QC: The Bell herbal tea did me a lot of good, it changed my life. I recommend it to anyone who like me was having trouble urinating. I noticed improvement from the first days. I continue to take it so good. I feel 100% better after a month. Thank you.

André Nadeau, 66, St-Anne de Sorel, QC: 10 years of calmed suffering! I have been taking Ezee Flow Herbal Tea for 4 months and I feel like a young man. Previously, I had tried remedies and medications that did not have much effect. I told many of my friends that they too were successfully cured. I am very satisfied. No side effects at all.

Where to get the product? You can have herbal tea at the following addresses:

NATURO HEALTH: Carrefour Saint-Georges; 8585, boul. Lacroix St-Georges Beauce, QC. CA G5Y 5L6 Phone: 418-228-9735.

New Life Health and Natural Health SPA: Phone: (243) 082 577 5588; Email: info@newlife-health.com

New Life Health and Natural health SPA: 256 avenue du Flambeau; Cheap Kinshasa. Tel: +243 81 388 7361 or Luano Avenue Num 3 Quado Kitambo, Kinshasa. Tel: +243 81 388 73611.

2-"Angels Secret" negative ion panty liner

The "Angels Secret" negative ion panty liner has been developed by JM Océan Avenue which is the union of two major multinational network marketing companies: Ocean Avenue and JM International. JM Océan Avenue is present in 5 continents and in almost 40 countries in the world and offers products that are ranked the best in the field of health and well-being.

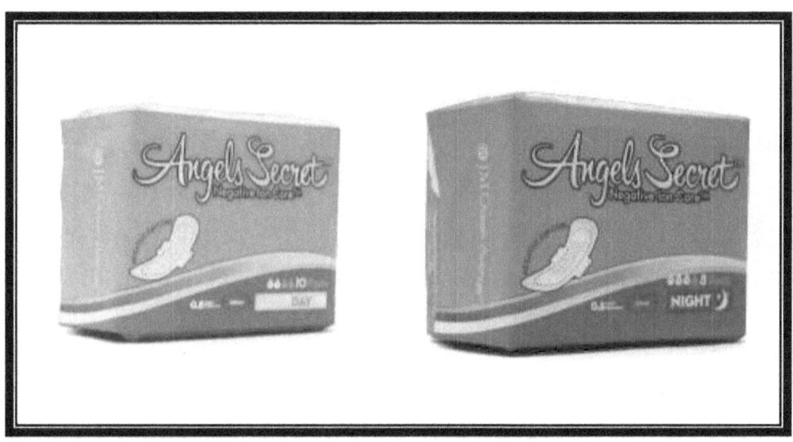

Figure 5: Secret Angels for Women on the Left, and for Men on the Right

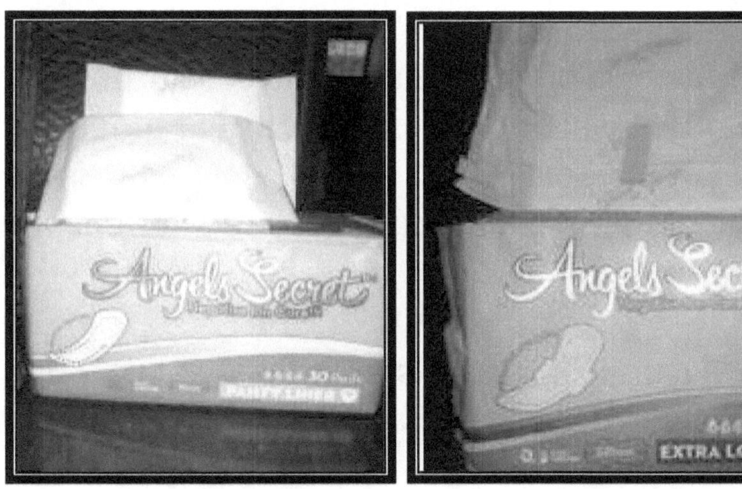

Figure N° 6: Intimate ladies' pads on the left and pant liners on the right.

Angels Secret can be used by women in the form of an intimate sanitary napkin, and by men in the form of panty liners.

It has a structure with seven protective layers, namely:

First layer: It is made of special cotton of high permeability allowing external drying and comfort.

Second layer: This is a band of anions that fights bacteria and inflammation and eliminates odors.

Third layer: This is a special water channel made of high quality cotton that prevents leaking liquids.

Fourth layer: This is a highly absorbent polymer that instantly absorbs women's menstrual blood.

Fifth layer: This is another special water channel designed to prevent leaks.

Sixth layer: It consists of a very tight polyethylene film membrane.

Seventh layer: This is a striated plastic adhesive.

Secret Angels used by men has major results:

It improves the libido and makes recover a strong erection ensuring harmonious, successful and satisfying sexual relations for both partners.

Indeed, BPH, by compressing the blood vessels of the penis of the man, makes it, during sexual stimulation, can no longer have a rigid penis and firm to penetrate the vagina of wife. Angels Secret restores this ability.

It fights various infections of the prostate and bladder. Because of the permanent retention of a certain residual amount of urine in the bladder because of the increased volume of the prostate, various bacteria develop and proliferate in this kind of culture broth that is the residual urine. It develops different germs that cause infections and inflammation of the prostate, as well as stones in the kidneys. The negative ions contained in the Angels Secret special band destroy all the germs contained in the urines of the bladder and that have begun to become embedded in the prostatic tissue.

It decreases the volume of the prostate: After 2 to 3 months of continuous use, a significant decrease in the volume of the prostate is observed, with its corollaries of ease of urination, decreasing the frequency of going to the toilet.

Secret Angels, used by women as an intimate towel, has the following properties:

It has a high absorption capacity: Particles made of super absorbent polymers guarantee an instant dry surface. Women are protected, with comfort, 24 hours a day.

It is highly breathable: Good ventilation is ensured by the use of materials that allow excellent air circulation.

The Natural Anion Strip releases nearly 6,000 anions per cm3 that kill bacteria and eliminate odors. In addition, these anions promote women's metabolism, strengthen blood circulation, regulate the menstrual cycle, restore hormonal balance and eliminate abdominal cramps, sources of painful menstruation for many women.

Contacts to join JM Ocean Avenue around the world and get Angels Secret

E-mail: nancymlmsuccess@gmail.com
Whatsapp: +221766186886
Skype: Martine Dems
Facebook: Nancy Mlm

For Europe or America, use the link below, put SN04285057 as in the box "Ambassador ID" and click "I agree" in the next page.
https://dist.jmtop.com/backOffice/bo/register?key

3-The phyto-drug ANTEPROST

Anterpost was developed in 2011, by Dr. Henri Charles Ainadou, director of S3P laboratories, on a scientific basis, from extracts of four plants native to Benin, namely: Caesalpinia bonduc (ADJIKWIN), Fagara xanthoxyloides (HETIN), Garcinia cola (AHOWETIN), Impera cylindrica. (SE SEKUN)

The Anterprost product has undergone clinical and therapeutic tests with patients who have been administered the product for 3 months.

The results of these tests were as follows:

- The volume of the prostate decreased by 30% in 55% of patients.
- PSA (prostate-specific antigen in French) decreased in 77.8% of cases.
- There was no toxicity to the liver and kidneys.

- There was a noticeable decrease in
urination difficulties, frequency of going to
the bathroom and a decrease in the amount
of residual urine.

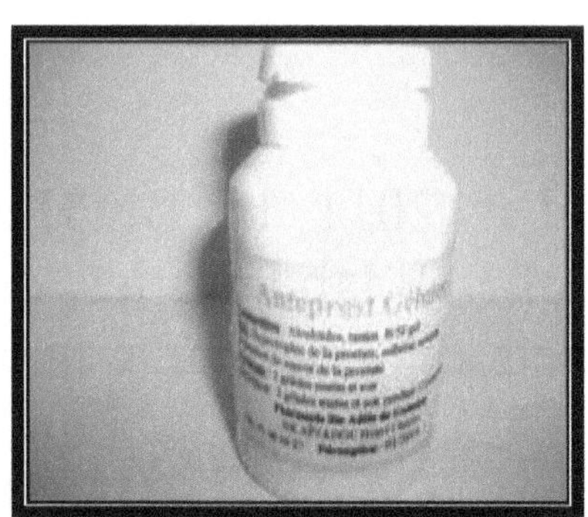 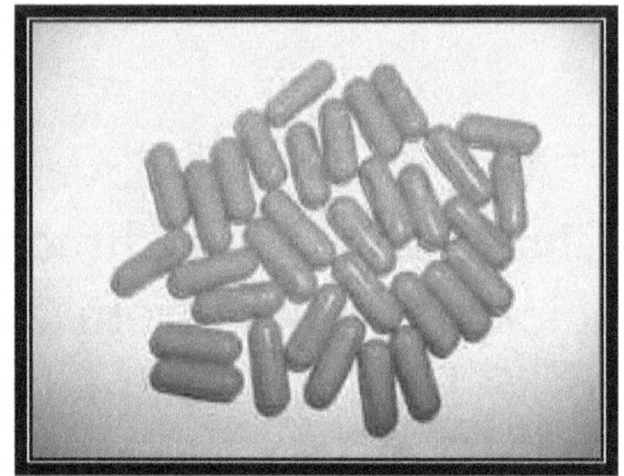

Figure N ° 7: The ANTERPROST product

Contacts: Dr. Henri Charles Ainadou; Saite
Adèle pharmacy; GODOMEY exchanger;
Cotonou; Benign.

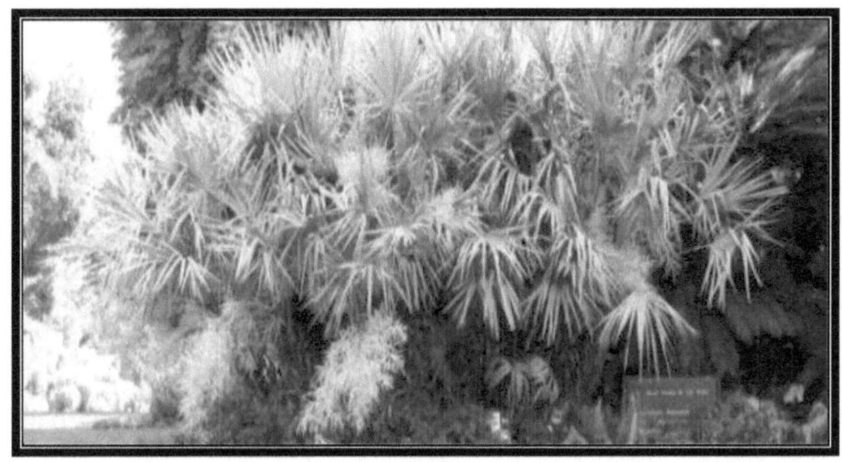

Figure N ° 8: The saw palmetto or serenoa repens

Serena repens is also called dwarf palm, or Florida palm, or saw palmetto, or saw palmetto, in English. Its fruits and berries contain carbon chain fatty acids, oil, beta sitosterol, phytosterol and anthranilic acids.

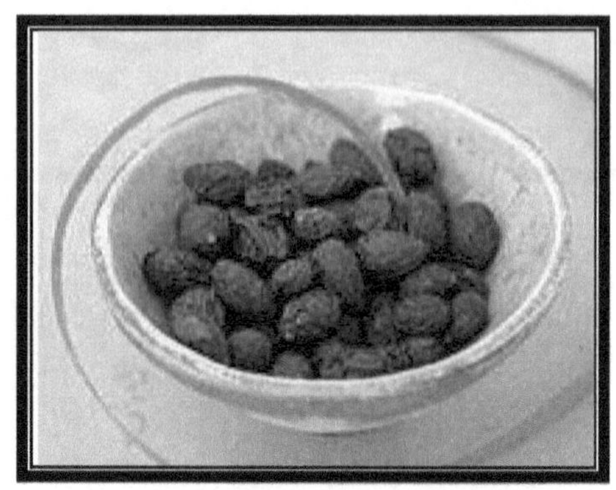

Figure N ° 9: The dwarf palm berries

The use of extracts of the saw palmetto, which is recommended to associate with extracts of nettle roots, relieves the difficulties of urination related to benign prostatic hypertrophy in phase I and II, as well as prostatitis chronic or inflammation of the prostate.

The recommended dosage is as follows:

- Standardized extract containing 85% to 95% of fatty acids and sterols: Take 160 mg twice daily.
- Standardized extract containing 25% fatty acids and sterols: Take 500 mg twice daily.
- Combined standardized extract: Take a daily supplement containing 240 mg of

nettle extract and 320 mg of saw palmetto extract.

According to a recent study, the use of 320 mg dwarf palm extract per day reduces the symptoms of BPH by 50% after 8 weeks of use.

5 - The plum tree of Africa (Pygeum africanum)

The plum tree of Africa is called Pygeum africanum or Prunus africana. His English name is red stinkwood. It belongs to the Rosaceae family (Rosaceae.)

It is a tree up to 30 m tall, with elliptical and thick leaves, small white flowers and round and red fruits. Its trunk is about one meter in diameter. It grows in the rain forests of the mountains of central and eastern Africa, from 1,000 meters above sea level. Its bark has a pinkish red color and a bitter almond smell.

It contains a fatty acid lipid fraction, phytosterols, pentacyclic triterpenic acids and linear alkanols.

It is used to treat nocturnal pollakiuria and benign prostatic hypertrophy. It is a decongestant that reduces the urge to urinate and weakens the residual urinary volume. The ferulic acid contained in the bark helps to stop the accumulation of cholesterol.

It is the bark that is used in herbal medicine.

The treatment dosage is as follows:

- In standardized extract dosed with 14% triterpenes and 0.5% n-docosanol: take 100 mg once or twice, in cure of six to eight weeks.
- In capsules: take 4 capsules a day, to swallow apart from the meals.

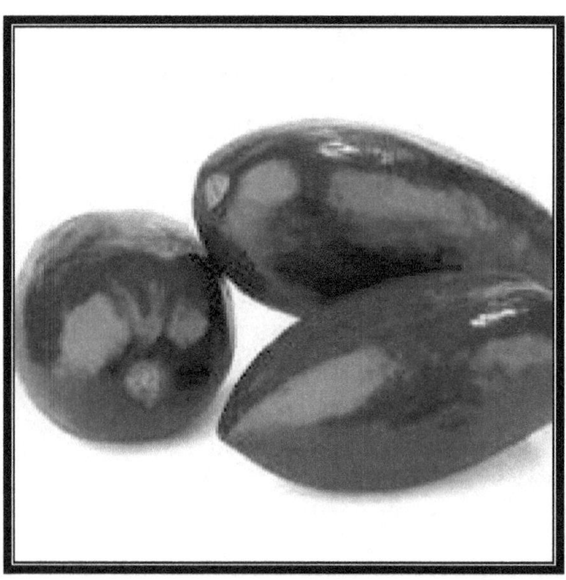

Figure N ° 10: The fruits of African plum

The big nettle is a perennial plant 60 to 150 cm high. It is completely covered with long stinging hairs or small soft bristles. The stems are erect; the leaves are lined with triangular teeth. The flowers are in clusters. The fruit is ovoid.

According to the common names, the plant is called nettle, dioecious nettle, nettle, stinging nettle, or common nettle. Its scientific name Urtica dioica. It belongs to the family Urticaceae (Urticaceae).

Nettle root contains polysaccharides, plant sterols, terpene acids, fatty acids, lignans and polyphenols.

Nettle is diuretic, depurative, antirheumatic, anti-inflammatory, analgesic, antimicrobial, anti-ulcer, anti-anaemic, hepatoprotective, antioxidant, hypoglycemic, antiallergic, immunostimulant, hypotensive, tonic, galactogenic.

It relieves painful joints; comes in addition to traditional treatments for inflammatory diseases of the urinary tract; decreases renal lithiasis; regulates urination disorders related to BPH. It is used to treat symptoms of the lower urinary system associated with benign prostatic hypertrophy. She also has anti-inflammatory and hypotensive actions.

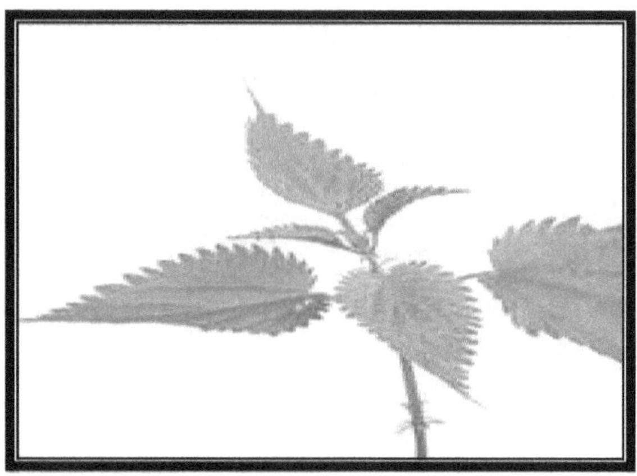

Figure N ° 11: The big nettle

The dosage of use is as follows:

- In root tea: Boil for ten minutes 1.5 g of powdered roots in cold water. Infuse for ten minutes and filter.
- In infusion of leaves: boil 3 tablespoons of dried leaves in 500 ml of water. Drink several cups a day of this preparation.
- Nebulosity (100 mg / capsule): take 2 capsules, three times a day.
- In decoction of roots, against the mictionnels disorders: to boil for three

minutes 50 g of roots in 1 liter of water. Infuse for twenty minutes. Drink at will.

Rye is a biennial herbaceous plant. Its scientific name is secale cereal. It belongs to the family Poaceae (grasses). It grows on cold and poor land. It is a large grass, with a height of up to 1.5 m for some varieties. His ear is bearded and looks like wheat. Spikelets have two seeds whose lemmas open when the grain matures.

Rye blossom pollen greatly affects the prostate. It relieves the symptoms of BPH, heals prostatitis and enlarges the prostate. It helps to relax the muscle of the bladder and the one surrounding the urethra to facilitate the passage of urine. It has ant-mutagenic activity on prostate cells, would reduce the toxic effects of cadmium, a likely inducer of hyperplasia. It reduces the size of the prostate by counterbalancing the level of dihydrotestosterone (DHT).

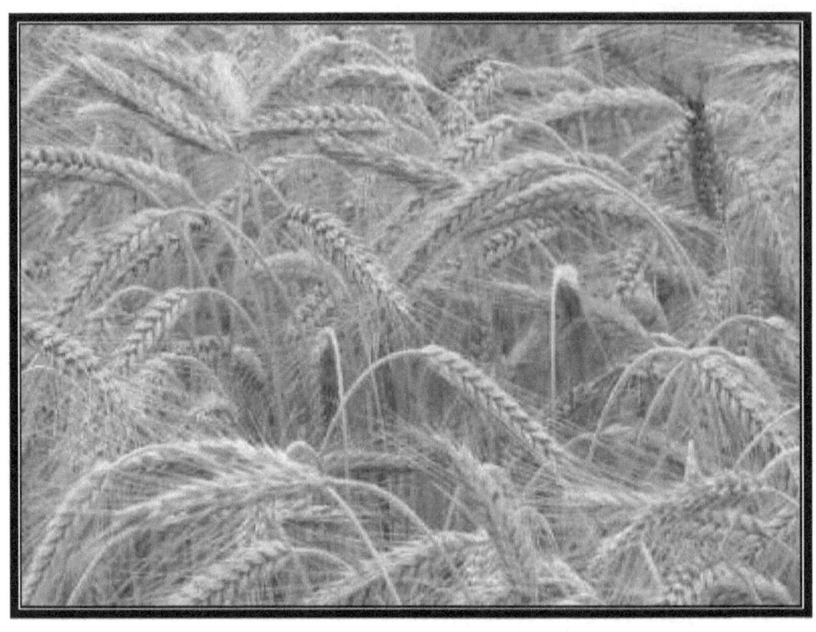

Figure N ° 12: The ears of rye or Secale cereal

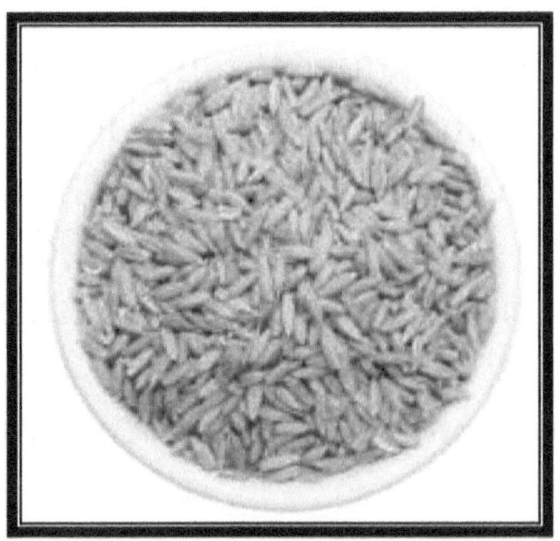

Figure N ° 13: Rye seeds

The Fireweed is a perennial herbaceous plant of the genus Chamerion and the family Onagraceae. It grows in all the temperate zones of the northern hemisphere. The stem can reach 0.5 to 2.5 m in height, the root is creeping and the leaves are numerous but not dense, alternate, sessile, whole, lanceolate and very elongated. The flowers are large and bright pink-purple, with 4 petals spread cross, a little uneven. The 8 stamens and style are curved down. The fruit is a linear red-brown capsule full of seeds, which opens with cracks at the top.

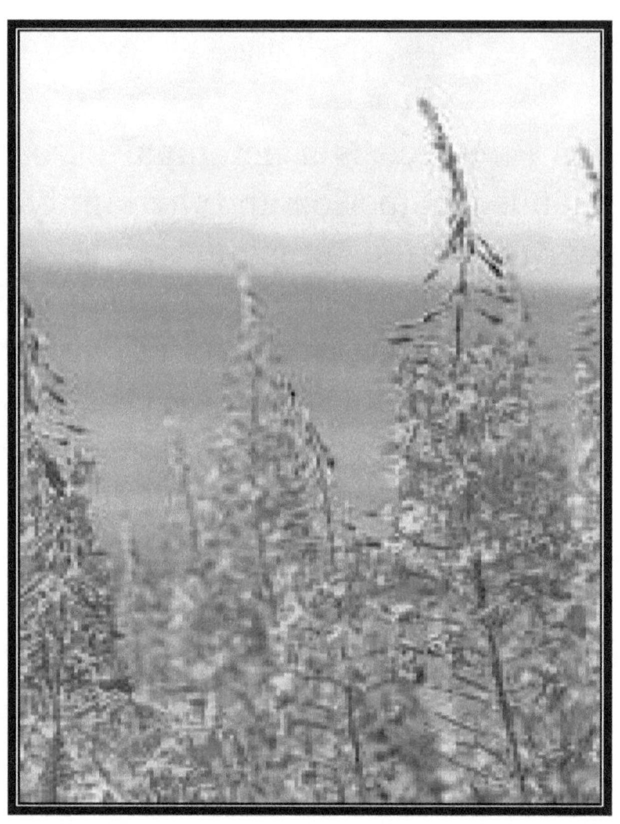

Figure N ° 14: Fireweed in ears

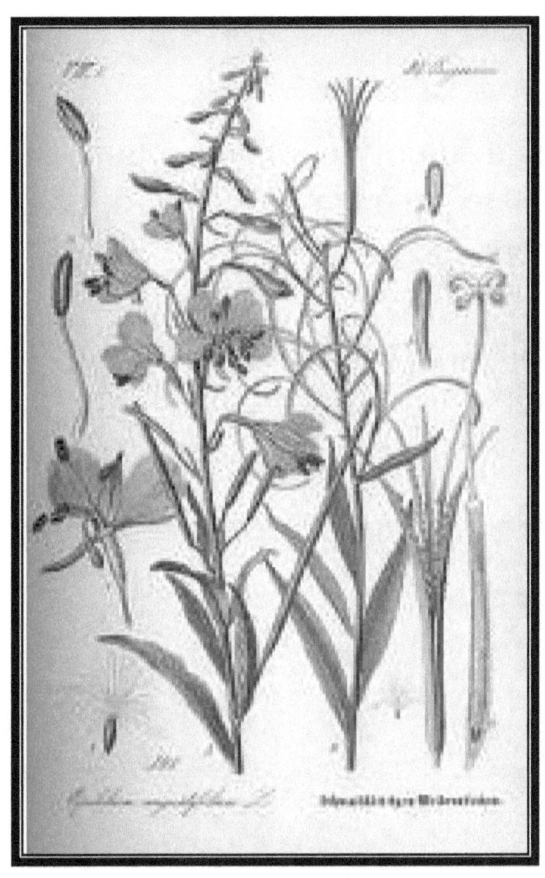

Figure N ° 15: Botanical Plate of Epilobium angustifolium

These are the leaves that are used in phyto-therapeutics. These leaves are available in herbalists. We recommend 30 g per liter of boiling water, to drink during the day.

Flax is a dicotyledonous plant of the family Linaceae. He is from Eurasia. It is grown for its textile fibers and oilseeds.

Flaxseeds are rich in alpha-linolenic acid (ALA), which helps to protect the body against many diseases.

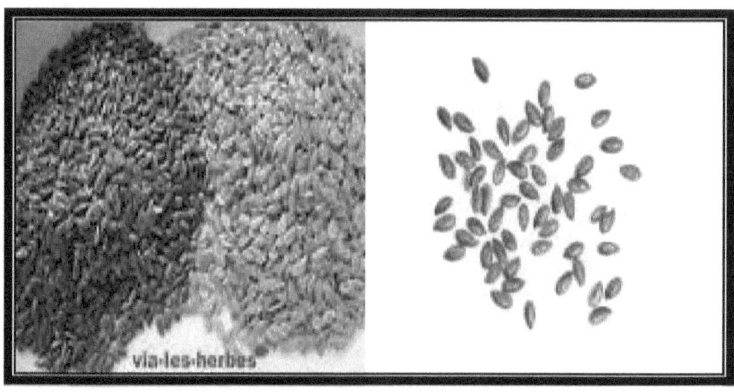

Figure N ° 16: Flax seeds

The consumption of flaxseed, given their high omega 3 content, protects the body against heart disease and arthritis. These seeds could also reduce the risk of breast cancer due to one, especially through the transformation of linseed lignans into estrogen-like molecules. Rich in soluble fiber, flaxseed is indicated to prevent constipation. On the other hand, flax seed has antioxidant properties, which is interesting for losing weight. Indeed, omega 3 flaxseed are fat burners and provide a natural laxative effect.

In addition to all these benefits, flaxseeds, with the lignans they contain, improve urinary symptoms after several months of consumption.

The dosage is as follows:

The flaxseed must be grinded before eating. The sheaths once ground, can be consumed 2 to 3 times a day, with plenty of water, before meals, using a tablespoon as a measure. Crushed flax seeds can also be added to soup, salad, gratin and even pastry.

Flaxseed oil, which contains about 7 g of alpha-linolenic acid per 15 ml tablespoon, can be eaten once or twice daily.

CONCLUSION

The treatment of benign prostatic hypertrophy by plants is clearly advantageous compared to conventional treatments because it has better efficacy, lower cost, and fewer side effects.

However, among all these proposed plants, it is difficult to determine which solution will be most effective if you suffer from BPH. Experience has shown that it is better to combine several plants or substances to achieve a significant improvement in symptoms. We must therefore focus on supplements that include a set of active substances.